Read a Bit! Talk a Bit! is a series of reading activity books intended for people with dementia and Alzheimer's disease. The books start with a short article or story for the participants to read, followed by a number of questions for the facilitator to ask. These questions are formulated to engage the participants in conversation and to encourage personal and meaningful reminiscences to flow.

All the reading pages are in large type, 44 pt, and the text is only on one page per spread in order to help the individual to concentrate on the text and to minimize the constraints of visual impairment.

Memories recalled from earlier in life are often very therapeutic for people with dementia. They provide opportunities for positive and meaningful engagement with the past. Remembering increases self esteem and a feeling of positive worth as the participants recall personal experiences

These fifteen books successfully achieve this thanks to the range of familiar topics and questions to prompt and encourage discussions.

Mary Morris is a diversional therapist and Gunilla Denton Cook is the author of the acclaimed book Lost Words. Drawing on their knowledge and experience they have collaborated on this series of activity books.

Read a Bit! Talk a Bit! Titles available

At the Movies	**Safety pin**
Cake	**Sandwich**
Chickens	**Scissors**
Garden	**Soup**
Lawnmower	**Stamps**
Money	**Teddy Bear**
Pencil	**Telephone**
Perfume	

Published by:
Denton Cook Pty Ltd
15 Elabana Cr.
Castle Hill NSW 2154
Australia

Phone +61 2 9651 3558
Fax   +61 2 9651 3007
dentoncook@bigpond.com
www.readabittalkabit.com

Someone said you can never be too thin or have too much money.

That may be the case for some.

Pass to next reader

1

Written by Gunilla Denton Cook and Mary Morris.
©2010 Denton Cook Pty Ltd

Money has been around for a long time.

The first coins are believed to have been stamped in Turkey in 650 BC.

Pass to next reader

Written by Gunilla Denton Cook and Mary Morris.

We work and are paid a salary for our efforts.

With this money we buy the food that we need to be able to work and earn more money.

Pass to next reader

3

Written by Gunilla Denton Cook and Mary Morris.
©2010 Denton Cook Pty Ltd

Farmers grow food which they sell at the market and receive payment for their goods.

This hasn't changed since the dawn of time.

Pass to next reader

4

Written by Gunilla Denton Cook and Mary Morris.
©2010 Denton Cook Pty Ltd

Manufacturers of different items do the same.

We all do what we are good at. We sell our wares or services to make the modern society function.

Pass to next reader

5

Written by Gunilla Denton Cook and Mary Morris.
©2010 Denton Cook Pty Ltd

Different countries have different currencies.

The majority of the European countries have agreed to all have the same currency.

6

Written by Gunilla Denton Cook and Mary Morris.
©2010 Denton Cook Pty Ltd

This makes it easier for everyone to trade across country borders.

In 2002 the Europeans changed from their old currencies to the Euro.

Pass to next reader

7

Written by Gunilla Denton Cook and Mary Morris.
©2010 Denton Cook Pty Ltd

Great Britain elected to keep using their Pounds and Pence.

The countries Sweden, Norway, Iceland and Denmark also kept their old currency Kronor.

Switzerland was another country to maintain their old currency the Swiss franc.

Pass to next reader

9

Written by Gunilla Denton Cook and Mary Morris.
©2010 Denton Cook Pty Ltd

The currency in the United States of America is the US dollar.

In Australia the currency is the Australian dollar.

Pass to next reader

10

Written by Gunilla Denton Cook and Mary Morris.
©2010 Denton Cook Pty Ltd

Money makes the world go around is another saying.

pass to group leader

11

Written by Gunilla Denton Cook and Mary Morris.
©2010 Denton Cook Pty Ltd

Questions

1. Does money make the world go round?

2. How much did a loaf of bread cost when you were young?

3. Did you save money in your youth?

4. Did your parents give you money for things or pocket money?

5. Did you keep your savings in the mattress?

6. What was the first thing you saved up for?

7. Can you remember how much your first house was?

8. What currency do they use in Europe?

9. What currency do they use in Great Britain?

10. Do you know what kind of money they use in Australia?

11. Can you remember how much was in your first pay check?

12

12. What did you do to earn your first pay check?

13. How did you get the money? In cash, as a check or deposited into the bank?

14. Did you put money in the bank?

15. Did you have a bank book?

16. If you didn't have enough money at the time to buy something what did you do? Save, use a credit card or get a loan?

17. Can you think of some proverbs related to money?

    Civility costs nothing.
    You can be poor, but honest.

18. What did you do when times were tough?

19. Who was the person who controlled the money in your family?

Written by Gunilla Denton Cook and Mary Morris.
©2010 Denton Cook Pty Ltd